DRUGS & CONSEQUENCES

THE TRUTH ABOUT INHALANTS

G. S. PRENTZAS

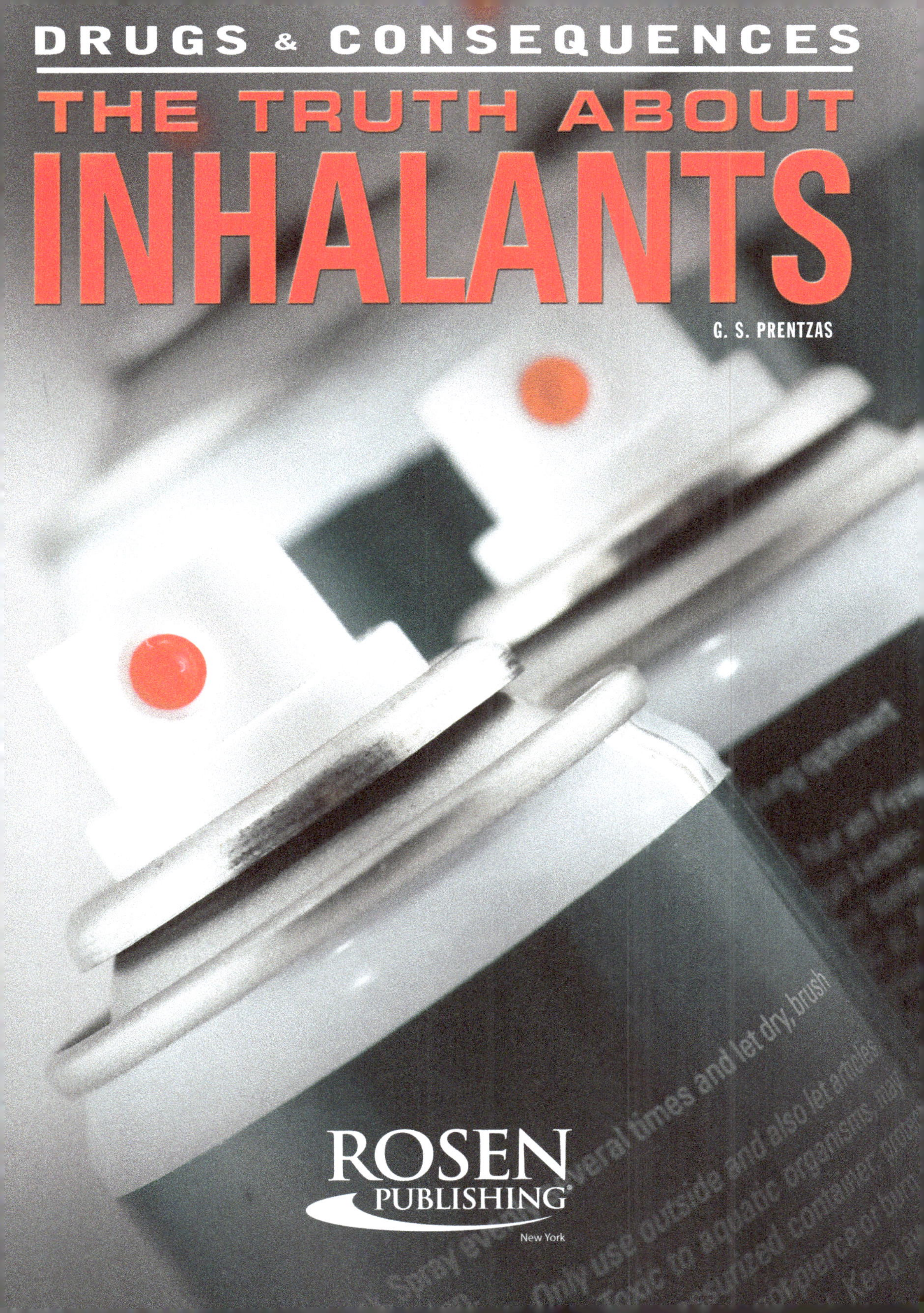

ROSEN PUBLISHING
New York

Published in 2014 by The Rosen Publishing Group, Inc.
29 East 21st Street, New York, NY 10010

First Edition

Library of Congress Cataloging-in-Publication Data

Prentzas, G. S.
The truth about inhalants/G. S. Prentzas.—First edition.
pages cm.—(Drugs & consequences)
Includes bibliographical references and index.
ISBN 978-1-4777-1893-3 (library binding)
1. Inhalant abuse—Juvenile literature. 2. Solvents—Health aspects—Juvenile literature. 3. Substance abuse—Prevention—Juvenile literature. I. Title.
RC568.S64P74 2014
616.86—dc23

2013018667

Manufactured in the United States of America

CPSIA Compliance Information: Batch #W14YA: For further information, contact Rosen Publishing, New York, New York, at 1-800-237-9932.

CONTENTS

INTRODUCTION

Inhalants are common chemical products found in homes, schools, and workplaces. Although these products serve a variety of useful purposes, some people misuse them as recreational drugs. They intentionally inhale the vapors that these products give off to experience a "high" or a "buzz." The inhaled chemicals quickly enter a person's bloodstream and produce a variety of temporary intoxicating effects. The term "recreational drug" is applied to a drug or substance that is used nonmedically for personal pleasure.

Many young people think inhalants cause no harm because many of the products used as inhalants are everyday items bought by their parents, sold in stores, and even advertised on television. The chemicals in the inhalant vapors, however, are poisons. They can change the way the brain works and harm other parts of an inhalant user's body. Once a person starts using inhalants, it can become a habit that is difficult to break. In some cases, the physical damage caused by habitual inhalant use is permanent. Inhalants users also experience other problems, such as failing grades, losing friends, and causing conflicts within their families.

Inhalant use is nothing new. People in ancient Egypt, China, and other places around the world inhaled the fumes from incense, oils, spices, and

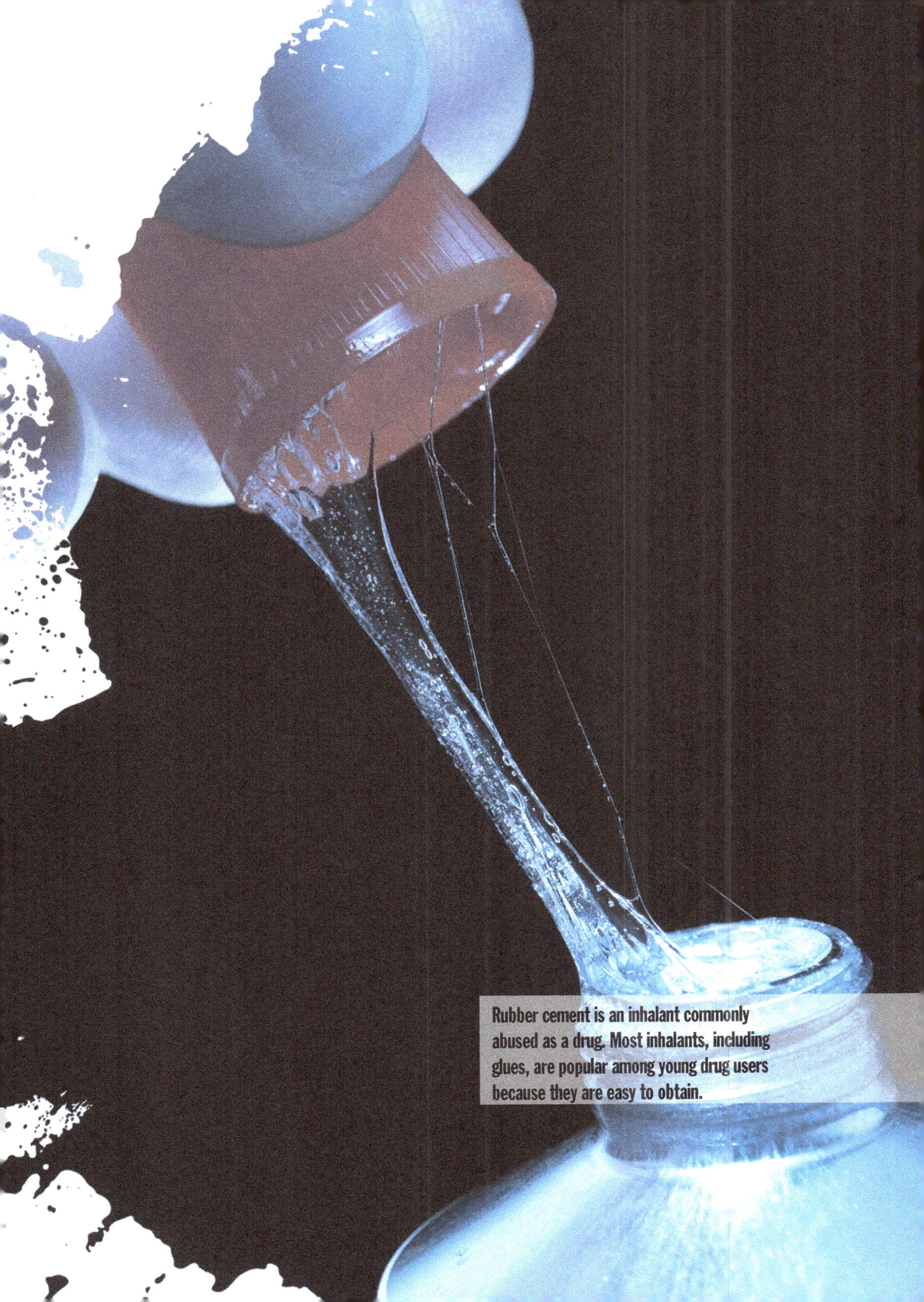

Rubber cement is an inhalant commonly abused as a drug. Most inhalants, including glues, are popular among young drug users because they are easy to obtain.

other substances as part of religious ceremonies or to experience their mind-altering effects. In the early 1800s, some people used ether and other anesthetics to get high. The use of inhalants in North America grew in popularity in the 1950s, and by the 1960s, it had become increasingly widespread among teenagers.

In 2012, the National Institute on Drug Abuse (NIDA) released its annual *National Survey on Drug Use and Health*. This report provides statistics on the abuse of many types of drugs. NIDA estimated that in 2011, nearly 1.9 million young people between the ages of twelve and seventeen in the United States had abused inhalants at least once during their life. A NIDA-sponsored study, *Monitoring the Future: National Results on Drug Use*, shows that 6 percent of eighth graders, 4 percent of tenth graders, and 3 percent of twelfth graders used an inhalant at least once during 2011.

Although inhalant abusers do not fit any specific profile, researchers have identified several characteristics that are common among young people who use inhalants. Both males and females use inhalants, but about twice as many young males in the United States have used inhalants than females. Although abusers come from all social and economic backgrounds, as well as all geographical regions, young people who live in poverty, experience child abuse at home, and perform poorly at school are more likely to abuse inhalants.

Abusers tend to start using inhalants in elementary or middle school and usually shift their drug use to other substances as they progress through high school. Users in different age groups generally prefer specific inhalants over others. New users of inhalants, who are typically between the ages of twelve and fifteen, most often sniff glue, lighter fluid, shoe polish, and spray paints. Teenagers who are sixteen and seventeen favor nitrous oxide. Nitrites usage is more prevalent among older teens and adults. Except for nitrites, the use of inhalants is uncommon among older teens and adults. Inhalants are the only type of drug that younger teens abuse more than older teens.

CHAPTER 1

A TOXIC HIGH

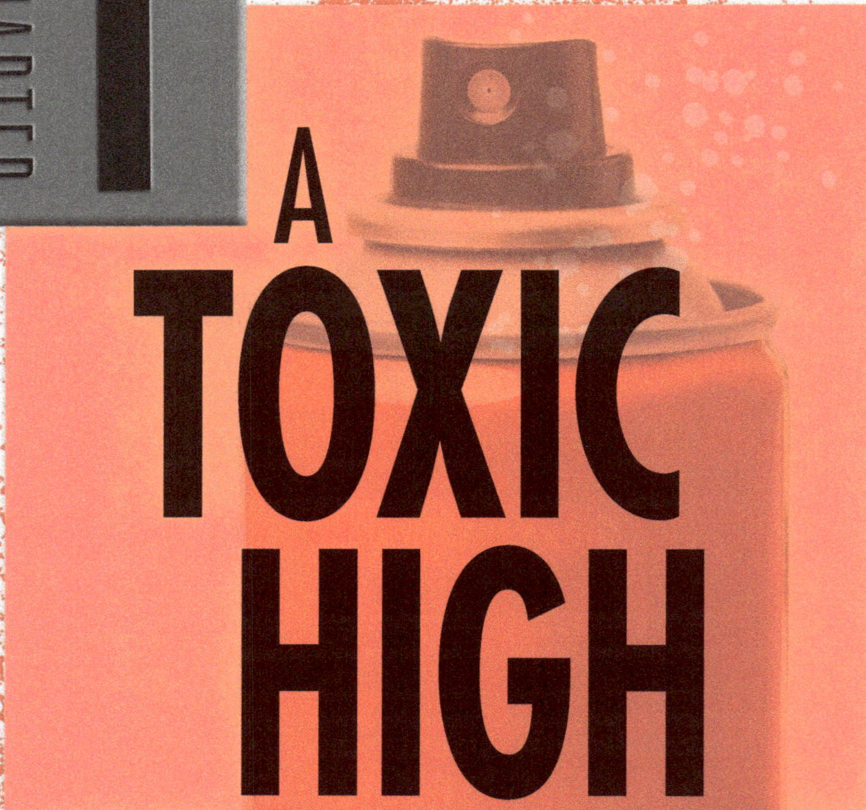

Many household and industrial products contain chemicals that have mind-altering properties when they are inhaled. Glues, markers, butane lighters, and cleaning fluids are common examples. These products are not made or sold to be taken as drugs. Because they have practical, everyday uses, most adults and young people do not consider these products as drugs. Some people use them, however, to get high.

When used as recreational drugs, these products are known as inhalants. Most people who use inhalants are young. Some drugs,

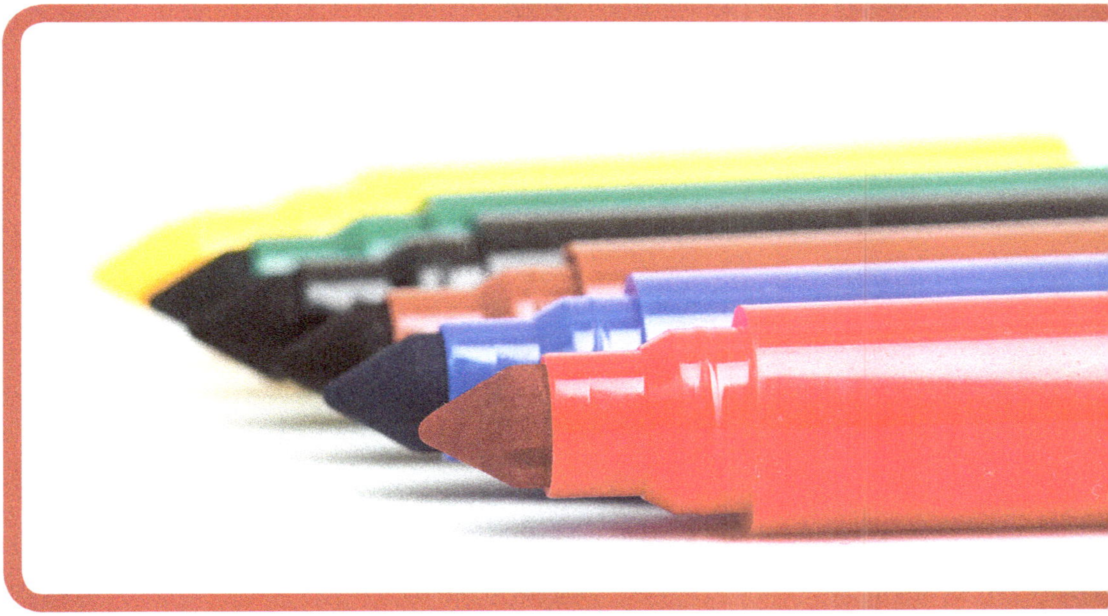

Uncapped felt-tip markers release vapors containing toxic chemicals. Although markers are meant to be used for writing and illustrating, some young people inhale their vapors to experience a quick, cheap high.

particularly cocaine, are sometimes inhaled. These drugs are not considered inhalants, though. The term "inhalants" refers to substances that are used only by inhaling. They are never abused by swallowing, injecting, smoking, or any other method.

Types of Inhalants

Inhalants are chemical substances that produce small particles of gas or mist, known as vapors. When they are inhaled into the lungs, these vapors produce a physical effect on the brain and other parts of the body. The effects produced by individual

THE HARMFUL CHEMICALS IN POPULAR INHALANTS

All inhalants contain toxic chemicals that cause damage to the brain, organs, and other parts of the body. Here are the harmful chemicals contained in popular types of inhalants:

Aerosols	
Spray paints	butane, fluorocarbon, toluene
Hair sprays	butane, propane, fluorocarbon
Air fresheners	butane, propane, fluorocarbon
Anesthetics	
Gas	nitrous oxide
Liquid	enflurane, halothane
Local	ethyl chloride
Cleaning Products	
Degreasers	tetrachoroethylene, trichloroethane, trichloroethylene
Spot removers	tetrachoroethylene, trichloroethane
Gases	
Dessert-topping cans	nitrous oxide
Nitrites	
Poppers	amyl nitrite, isobutyl nitrite, butyl nitrite
Solvents	
Correction fluid	toluene, methylene chloride, methanol
Lighters and lighter fluid	butane, isopropane
Nail polish remover	acetone
Paint thinners	toluene, methylene chloride, methanol

inhalants differ. An inhalant may make the user temporarily lightheaded, happy, excited, or agitated. A variety of products contain chemicals that produce physical effects when they are inhaled. These products can be categorized into four groups.

Volatile Solvents

Volatile solvents are liquids that vaporize, or turn to a gas or mist, at usual indoor temperatures. If you have smelled the strong odor of gasoline or rubber cement, you know what a volatile solvent is. What you smelled are the vaporized chemicals that are in these

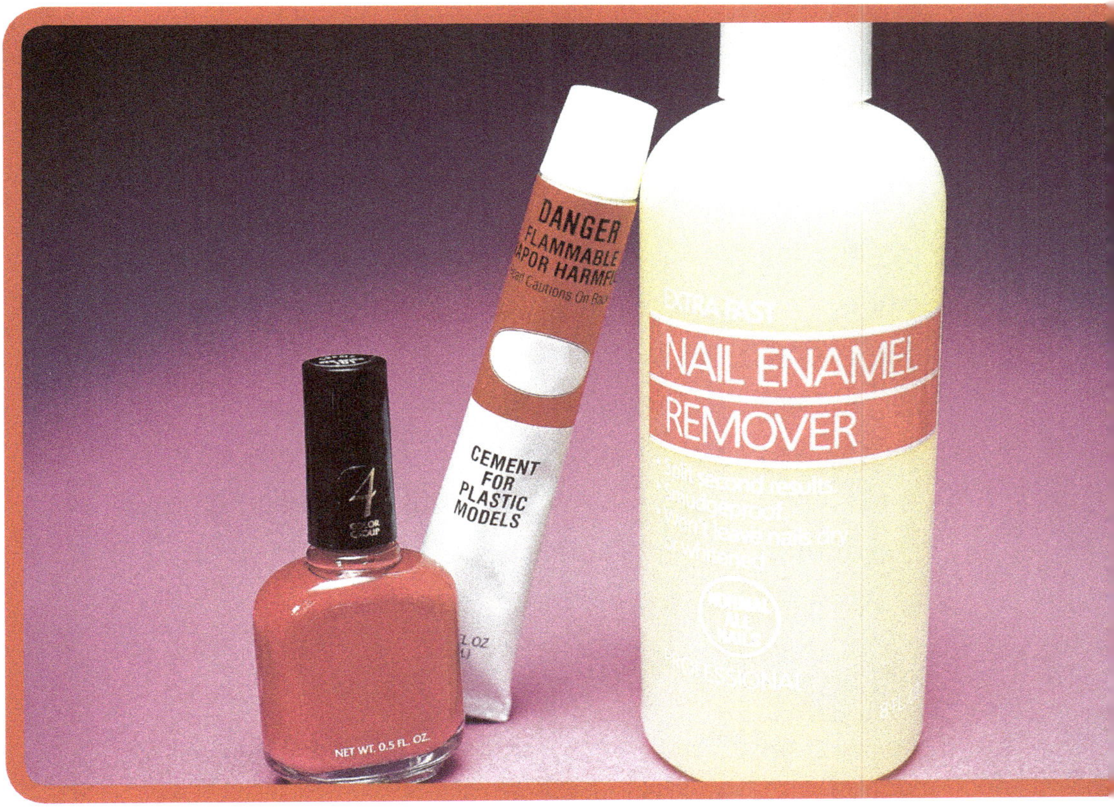

Nail polish, glue, and nail polish remover are volatile solvents. Many parents, teachers, and young people do not realize that these familiar products are sometimes abused as drugs.

substances. Many common household and industrial products are volatile solvents, including nail polish remover, gasoline, and paint thinner. Some school and office supplies—including glue, felt-tip markers, and correction fluids—are also volatile solvents.

Gases

Gases are substances that are neither a solid nor a liquid. For instance, air is a type of gas. Some common products contain gases that people abuse as inhalants. The gases in butane lighters, propane tanks, and helium balloons are examples of gas inhalants.

Gases used as medical anesthetics are also sometimes utilized as inhalants. An anesthetic is a substance that makes a person lose feeling or consciousness. Doctors employ anesthetics to perform surgery, dental work, and other medical procedures so that patients do not feel pain. Nitrous oxide, ether, and chloroform are common anesthetics. Nitrous oxide, or laughing gas, is the gas most often abused as an inhalant. It is used in some products as a propellant, a gas that expels the contents of a container. Users typically inhale nitrous oxide from cans of supermarket whipped cream. They also inhale nitrous oxide from small gas cartridges used in whipped cream dispensers.

Aerosols

Aerosols are sprays that contain solvents. Aerosols used as inhalants include many types of common household items.

Spray paints, hair sprays, and some computer cleaning products are examples of aerosol inhalants.

Nitrites

Nitrites are compounds that belong to the alkyl nitrite chemical group. Their medical uses include reviving an unconscious person and treating heart pain. Amyl nitrite, butyl nitrite, and isopropyl nitrite are the most common types of nitrites abused as inhalants. The federal government limits the sale of nitrites. Most people need a prescription to buy them. Despite this restriction, nitrites are sold in small bottles often labeled as video head cleaner, room odorizer, or liquid aroma. Nitrites are often called "poppers" because users pop open a bottle of nitrites to inhale the chemicals inside.

Amyl nitrite is sometimes confused with amyl nitrate, which is in a different chemical family. Amyl nitrate is an ingredient in fuel additives, which are volatile solvents that are added to gas or other fuels to improve the performance of vehicle engines. Fuel additives are also used as inhalants, which leads to the confusion between these two similar-sounding chemicals.

Recreational Use

People who use inhalants breathe chemical vapors into their lungs through the nose or mouth. This process is often called "huffing." People use drugs, including inhalants, for many reasons. Some find drug use exciting. Others want to experience

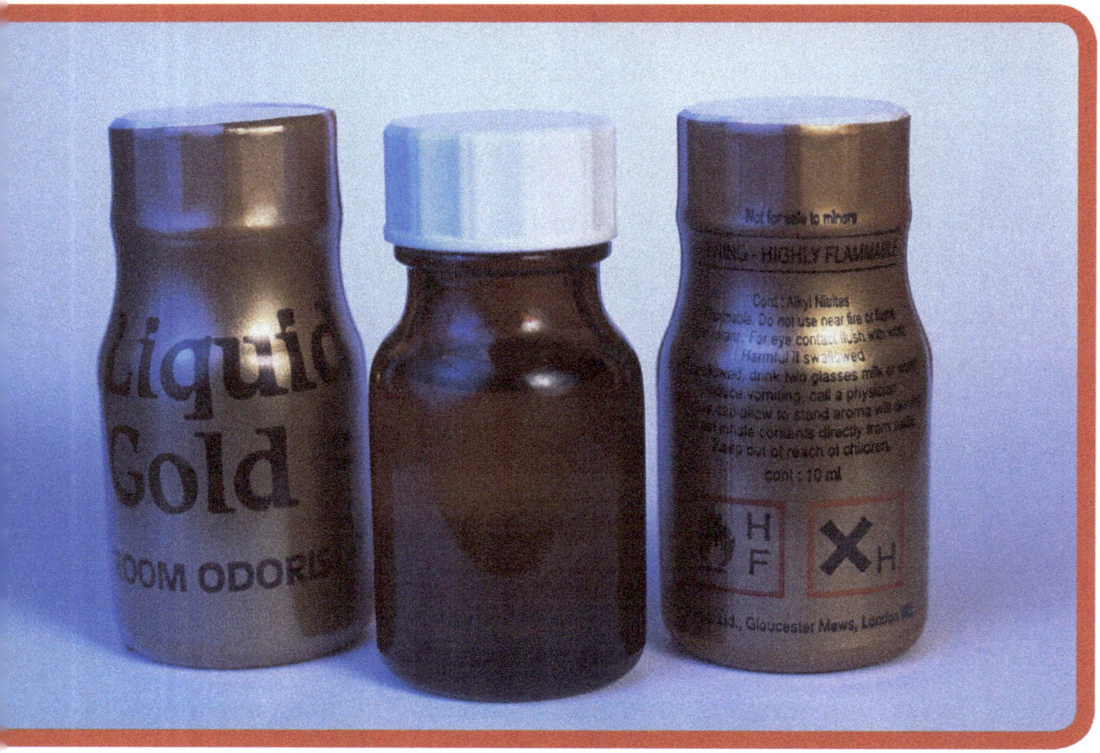

Liquid Gold is a brand of nitrites. Because a prescription is needed to buy nitrites legally in the United States, nitrites are sold in some stores in bottles labeled as "room deodorizers" or other products.

something new. Some inhalant abusers want to rebel against their parents or society or to escape the problems in their life. Others want to look cool or tough in front of friends or are trying to fit in with a group. Inhalant abuse often has a social aspect. Many young people use inhalants with friends or other inhalant users.

Drug abuse researchers have identified four different types of inhalant abusers. Some users are typically between the ages of ten and sixteen and have a short history of inhalant use. Some of these users usually take inhalants with friends, but others mostly use inhalants while they are alone. The other two types of users have a history of inhalant abuse exceeding five years. Habitual users are usually older, between the ages of twenty and twenty-three, and often use inhalants every day with friends. Some habitual users take inhalants by themselves. People in both groups who use inhalants habitually often have

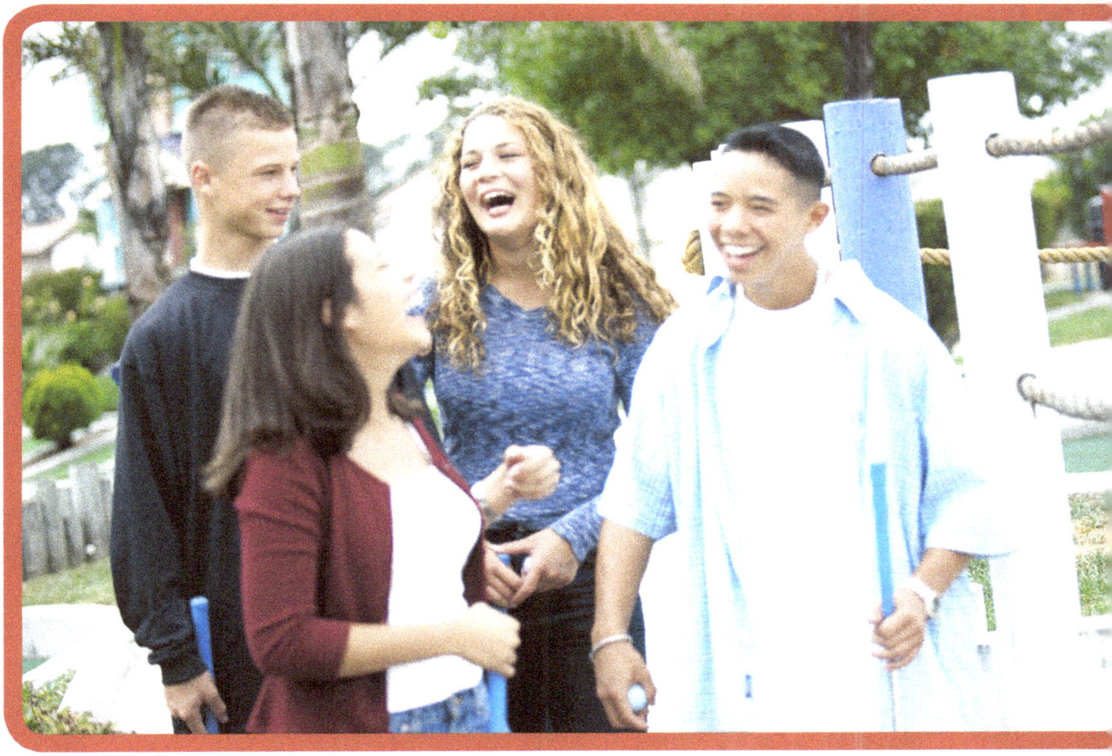

Inhalants are sometimes used among a group of friends, and a newcomer to a group may feel that he or she must try huffing to fit in. Researchers report that users who are between the ages of ten and sixteen generally don't use inhalants for a long period of time.

limited education and poor social skills, and they may have suffered permanent brain damage because of inhalants.

The Popularity of Inhalants

A variety of factors contribute to making inhalants popular substances to abuse among young people. Most abusers have easy access to the products used as inhalants. Unlike most other drugs, the substances used as inhalants have primary purposes other than producing a high. These products are easily found in homes, stores, workplaces, and other locations. A person abusing inhalants also has many different products to choose from. More than one thousand products can be abused as an inhalant. If a favored inhalant is not available, a user has many other options. Many of these substances are inexpensive or can be obtained for free in the home or at work. Younger drug users often do not have enough money to buy the drugs that are typically popular with older teens, such as alcohol and marijuana.

Many of the products used as inhalants are legal to buy and possess. Abusers often choose to use inhalants because they do not have to get them from a drug dealer. Abusers usually do not need to worry about the police catching them with the product. Although the sale of one category of inhalants—nitrites—is restricted nationwide, they are often sold in packages labeled as other products. This packaging makes it difficult for the police to enforce the law and keep nitrites off of store shelves. Laws in many states prohibit the sale of certain products that are used as inhalants, such as spray paint, to minors. Some stores do not obey these laws consistently, and law enforcement agents rarely catch stores selling the products to underage people because the police are routinely focused on more important crimes and issues. These laws are typically aimed at the merchants selling the products.

Underage purchasers in many states face no legal penalties when caught possessing a restricted product. Some states, however, have laws prohibiting the abuse of inhalants. For example, the Colorado Controlled Substances Act states, "No one shall knowingly smell or inhale the fumes of toxic vapors for the purpose of causing a condition of euphoria, excitement, exhilaration, stupefaction, or dulled senses of the nervous system." A young person caught using inhalants in Colorado and states with similar laws may face charges in juvenile court or regular criminal court, depending on his or her age. In Colorado, a second offense may lead to jail time.

Inhalant abusers do not need any paraphernalia, such as needles, rolling papers, or bongs, to get high. They usually simply inhale directly from a container. Using inhalants is also easier for abusers to conceal. Inhalant use can occur in many different places without attracting attention or taking a big risk of being caught. The high produced by inhalants does not last long, so users return to a normal state more quickly than if they get high on most other types of drugs. Inhalant use is also more difficult for parents, teachers, and friends to detect. Adults are also often unaware of the signs of inhalant use or how widespread inhalants abuse is among young people. Many young people do not know the serious consequences of using inhalants. Some drug education programs place an emphasis on more popular drugs. In addition, there are schools that do not provide any type of drug education or awareness programs.

CHAPTER 2

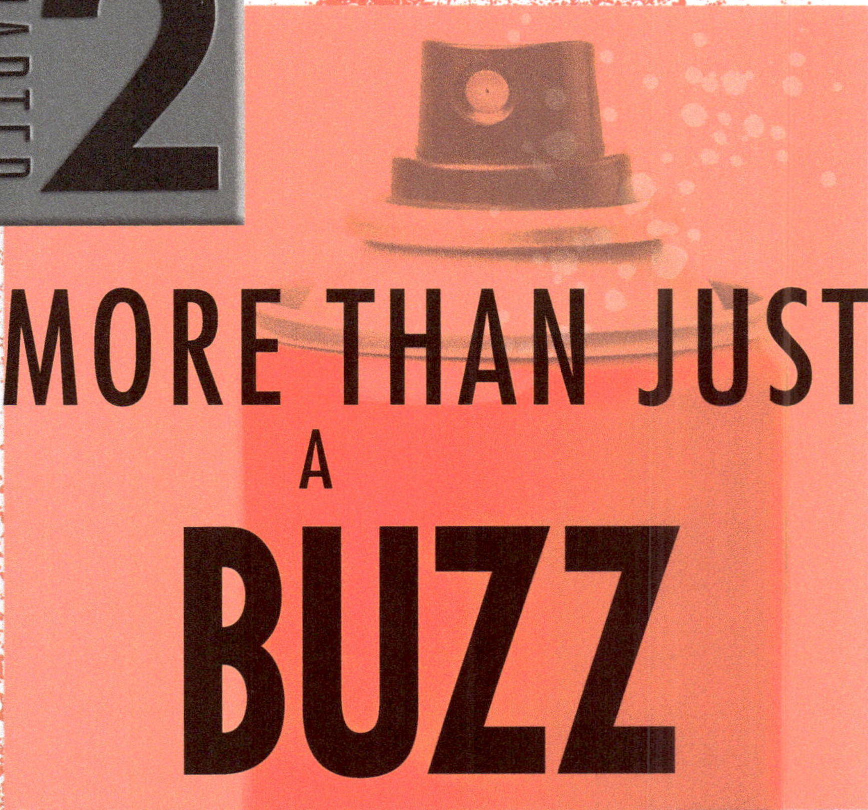

MORE THAN JUST A BUZZ

When a person inhales, oxygen and other gases fill the lungs. Each lung contains small tubes known as bronchioles, and at the end of these tubes are tiny air sacs, or alveoli. A web of small blood vessels called capillaries covers each air sac. The blood in these capillaries absorbs oxygen from the air sacs and carries it throughout the body. Oxygen is the fuel that all cells in the human body need to live and function. When the blood in capillaries surrounding the air sacs absorbs oxygen, it releases carbon dioxide back into the lungs at the same time. Carbon dioxide is a gas that cells in the body produce as they use oxygen. When a person exhales, the lungs expel carbon dioxide from the body.

When someone breathes in an inhalant, a similar exchange occurs in the lungs. An inhalant's vapors or gases enter the lungs, and their chemicals quickly enter the bloodstream. The heart distributes the blood—and the chemicals they contain—throughout the body, including to the brain and nervous system.

How the Brain and Nervous System Work

The brain is the most important organ in your body. It controls all of your thoughts, memories, feelings, senses, movements, and other body functions. Protected by the skull, the brain weighs only 3 pounds (1.4 kilograms). Despite its small size, it has many folds and grooves that contain more than one hundred billion nerve cells known as neurons. Neurons are a special type of nerve cell that uses electrical or chemical signals to send information throughout the body. Each neuron has tiny branches that connect to other neurons.

The nervous system carries messages between the brain and other parts of the body. The spinal cord is the main branch of the nervous system. This long bundle of nerves extends about 18 inches (46 centimeters) from the brain down through the spine. Thin strands of nerves are connected to the spinal

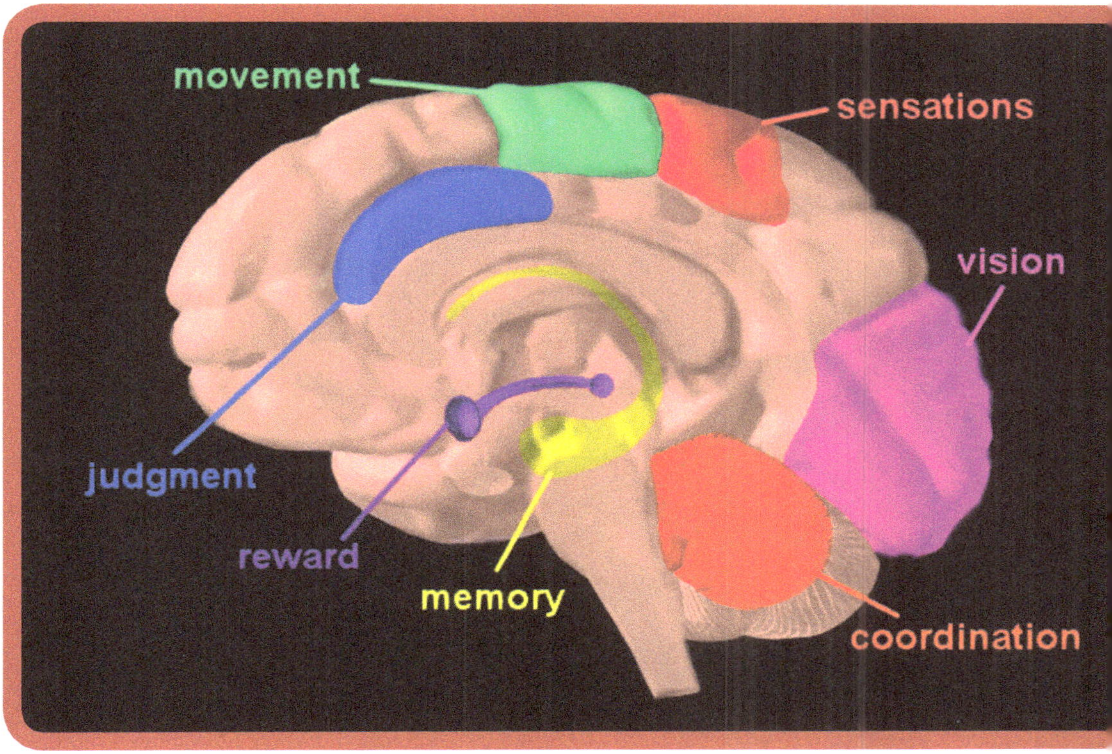

Inhalants have a variety of short-term effects on the brain. They may temporarily impair certain sections of the brain, including those that control coordination, vision, and memory.

cord along its entire length. These nerves shoot out, reaching every part of the body.

When a nerve in the body senses a change, it transmits an electrical impulse or chemical signal to the brain. The brain analyzes the information from the nerve and sometimes sends out a message that causes a response from the body. For example, when you grab a sharp object, nerves in your fingers and hand send pain messages to your brain. The brain analyzes these messages and quickly sends out a message to the muscles in your hand and arm to release the object.

Short-Term Impacts on the Brain

The most significant physical effects of inhalants occur in the brain. Soon after breathing in an inhalant, a user feels sensations similar to those produced by alcoholic beverages. Like alcohol, the chemicals in inhalants produce a short-term, or acute, change in the way the brain works. Most inhalants slow down the messages that the brain sends to the nervous system.

TOLUENE'S IMPACT ON THE NERVOUS SYSTEM

Habitual use of toluene—a chemical found in many inhalants, including correction fluid, paint thinner, and gasoline—damages the protective coating of fatty tissue that protects nerve fibers in the body's nervous system. This coating, known as myelin, surrounds nerve fibers in much the same way that plastic covers electrical wires. Toluene breaks up myelin, causing nerve fibers to malfunction. These fibers start sending messages more slowly or stop working completely. Research has shown that the destruction of nerve fibers caused by toluene is similar to the damage to the nervous system seen in people suffering from multiple sclerosis and other neurological disorders.

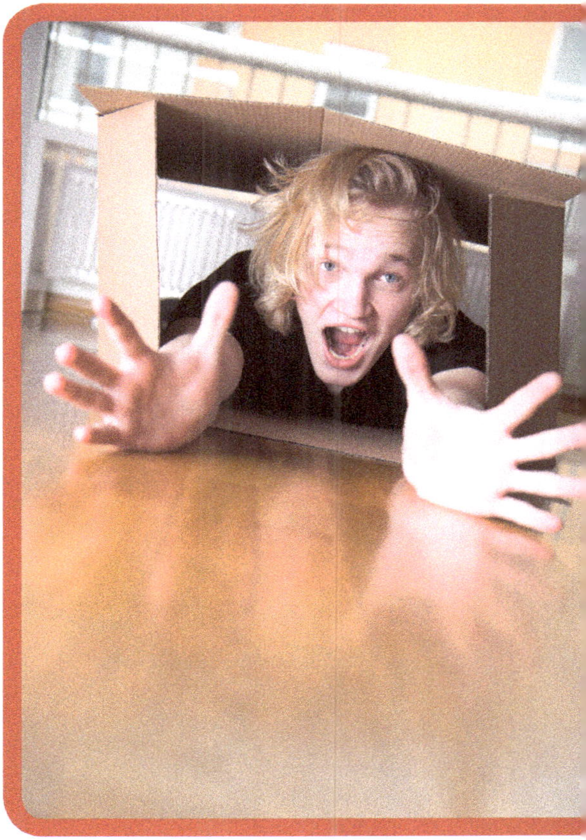

A teen jokingly plays jack-in-a-box. Some inhalants may make a person more outgoing or increase his or her sense of happiness and playfulness.

When a person uses an inhalant, the effects usually occur quickly. At first the user may feel happy, lightheaded, strange, or "out of it." The individual may later experience slurred speech or a lack of coordination. Slowed-down brain messages cause all of these effects.

Inhalants produce a euphoria that lasts anywhere from about two to twenty minutes. To keep the high going, users sometimes breathe in an inhalant again and again. Using an inhalant repeatedly in a short period may make the user less reserved or timid. Similar to the effects of being drunk on alcohol, the person may be more talkative and outgoing but less in control of his or her actions. Some inhalants make users sleepy or give them a headache that may last several hours.

Nitrites act on the brain differently from other types of inhalants. Instead of slowing down brain functions like most inhalants, they speed them up by temporarily causing an increase in the flow of blood to the brain. When it is inhaled, a nitrite relaxes most blood vessels in the body, causing them to expand slightly. The user's blood pressure falls briefly because the heart is circulating the same amount of blood through these enlarged blood vessels. To compensate for the sudden drop in blood pressure, the heart starts beating faster to bring the blood pressure back to its normal level. When the heart starts beating more quickly, an inhalant user starts feeling a sense of warmth, along with a pounding heart. The person's face and chest may also turn red as blood begins flowing faster through the body. The expansion of blood vessels in the brain causes pressure inside the brain to increase. This change in pressure, along with the increase in blood flow to the brain, usually causes a brief "rush" or period of happiness after nitrite use. The effects caused by nitrites usually wear off in about two minutes.

Long-Term Impacts on the Brain

Scientific research conducted on both animals and humans has shown that inhalants are toxic. Some of the chemicals in inhalants are eventually expelled in bodily waste. Other chemicals, however, remain in the body. Nerve cells and fatty tissues in the brain and central nervous system absorb these harmful chemicals. Chronic damage to the brain and nervous system is one of the major effects of the long-term use of inhalants. "Chronic" is a medical term meaning "long-lasting" or "permanent." Medical

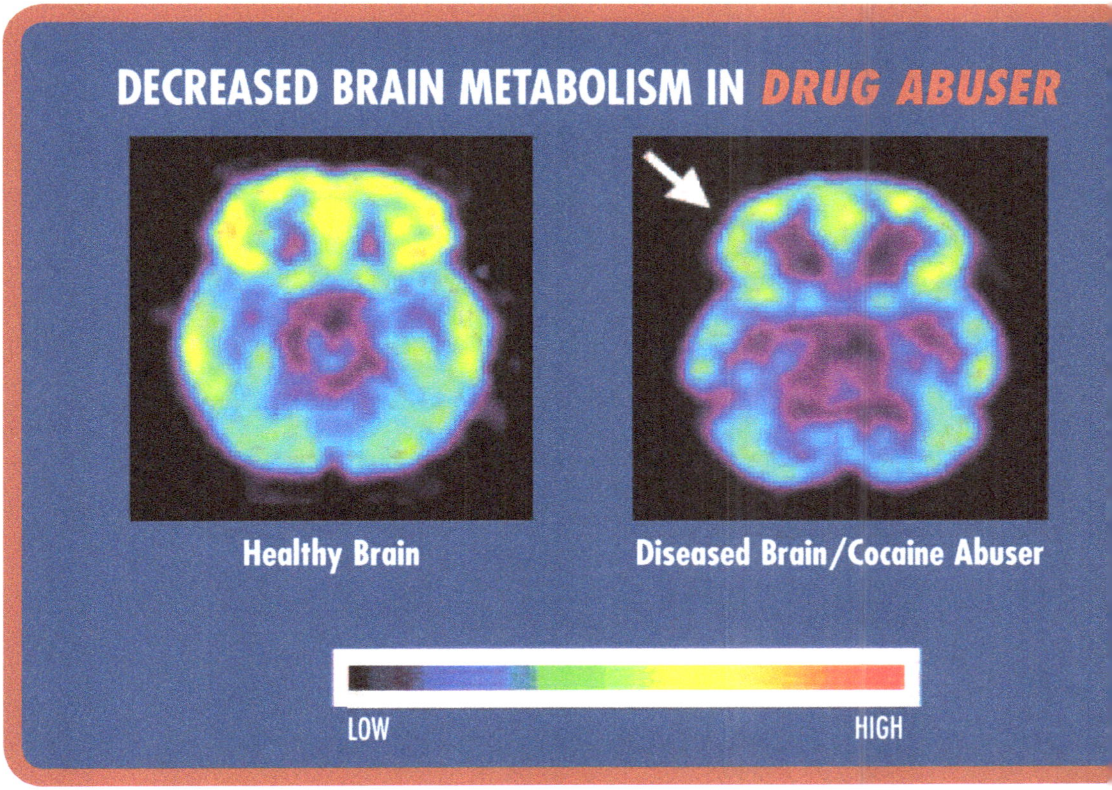

Brain scans show the difference in brain functioning between a healthy brain *(left)* and the brain of a cocaine addict *(right)*. Long-term inhalant abuse may result in similar damage to the brain.

researchers still do not know all of the effects that inhalants have on the brain and nervous system.

Prolonged use of inhalants can damage nerve cells in different parts of the brain. The chemicals in inhalants change the composition of the neurons in your brain. Neurons damaged by the use of inhalants slow down the electrical signals sent between the brain and nerves throughout the body.

Research has shown that long-term use of inhalants causes changes in a person's brain, reducing the size of some sections. If neuron damage due to inhalant abuse occurs in the prefrontal cortex, the part of the brain just behind the forehead, a person may struggle to focus attention, organize thoughts, solve problems, and make future plans. If the damage occurs in the cerebellum, which sits at the lower rear of the brain, a person may experience trouble with coordination and balance. He or she may move slowly or clumsily. Long-term inhalant use can also harm neurons in the hippocampus, an interior part of the brain. Damage to these neurons may affect a person's memory. The individual may be unable to learn new things or recognize familiar people or objects. Inhalants also affect neurons in the parts of the brain that control sight and hearing. A person may develop impaired vision or hearing and in some cases become blind or deaf from abusing inhalants.

MYTHS & FACTS

MYTH Inhalants are not addictive like other drugs.

FACT Inhalants can be addictive. Some users experience an intense urge to continue using an inhalant.

MYTH People use inhalants to deal with breathing problems.

FACT People who suffer from asthma and breathing problems use *inhalers*. These devices contain drugs prescribed by a doctor, usually either a type of steroid that eases irritation in the airways or a drug that enlarges the breathing passages. Inhalants are solvents, gases, or other substances that contain dangerous chemicals.

MYTH Using inhalants is safe.

FACT The chemicals in inhalants can harm your breathing passages and remain in your body for as long as two weeks after sniffing or huffing them. Long-term use can cause permanent damage to your brain, organs, and other parts of your body. An inhalant can also kill you, even if you are using it for the first time.

CHAPTER 3

THE DAMAGE DONE

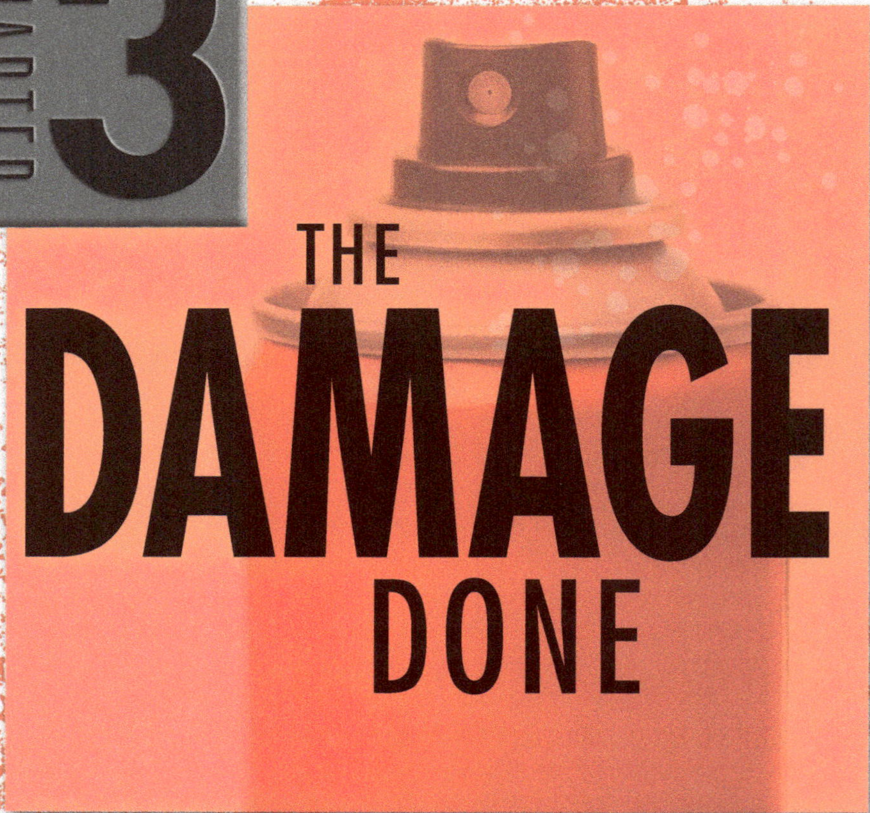

Besides affecting the brain and nervous system, inhalants have effects on many other parts of the body. The effects on the body are usually temporary, but serious consequences may occur after habitual use. Some of the effects of long-term inhalant use on the body may go away when a person stops using inhalants. Others are permanent. There is no safe way to use inhalants. Every time a person uses an inhalant, that individual risks injury or even death.

Acute Effects

When a person inhales a solvent or other inhalant, the chemicals in the substance enter the bloodstream through the lungs. The blood distributes the chemicals to cells throughout the body. The chemicals in inhalants may cause a variety of temporary effects on a person's body. The effects usually last for only a short time. If the inhalant is taken repeatedly, however, the effects may last several hours.

Most inhalants cause an increase in a user's heart rate. A user may experience a headache, pain in the abdomen, or nausea. The nausea sometimes results in vomiting. Numbness and tingling of hands or feet, muscle weakness, and limb spasms are other common physical effects associated with various inhalants. A user may also feel tired, his or her speech may be slurred, and the person may have trouble walking or performing other acts requiring coordination. The mood of a person using inhalants may swing from happy to sad, and he or she may even become violent. Inhalant users sometimes lose consciousness.

Chronic Effects

Over time, the toxic chemicals in inhalants build up in the body. Repeated use of inhalants may lead to a variety of long-term effects on the body. Using inhalants regularly may dry out the mucous membrane in a user's mouth and nose. Mucous

IN CASE OF AN INHALANT EMERGENCY

Inhalant use often leads to emergency medical situations. If you discover a friend or another person who is in a state of crisis after using an inhalant, it is important to remain calm and get help immediately. Take the following steps:

- Keep the person relaxed and comfortable. Calmness reduces stress on the heart, lowering the risk of heart failure due to inhalant use. In addition, if the person becomes agitated, he or she may become violent.
- Call 911 immediately to request emergency medical services.
- Open windows and doors to make sure the room is well ventilated.
- Determine which inhalant the person has used. This information will help medical personnel determine the best course of treatment.
- Call the American Association of Poison Control Centers' Poison Help Line for medical and other advice. Its twenty-four-hour, toll-free number is (800) 222-1222. You can also call the toll-free number on the label of the inhalant product for additional information.
- If the person stops breathing, perform CPR if you have the training.
- When medical assistance arrives, provide the essential information about the person's condition and the inhalant that was used.

membranes line internal organs and body cavities that are exposed to the air, such as the mouth and nose. Along with certain glands, some mucous membranes produce a thick fluid known as mucus. When mucous membranes dry out because of inhalants, users start to sneeze, cough, wheeze, or salivate excessively. They may also experience frequent nose bleeds due to dry

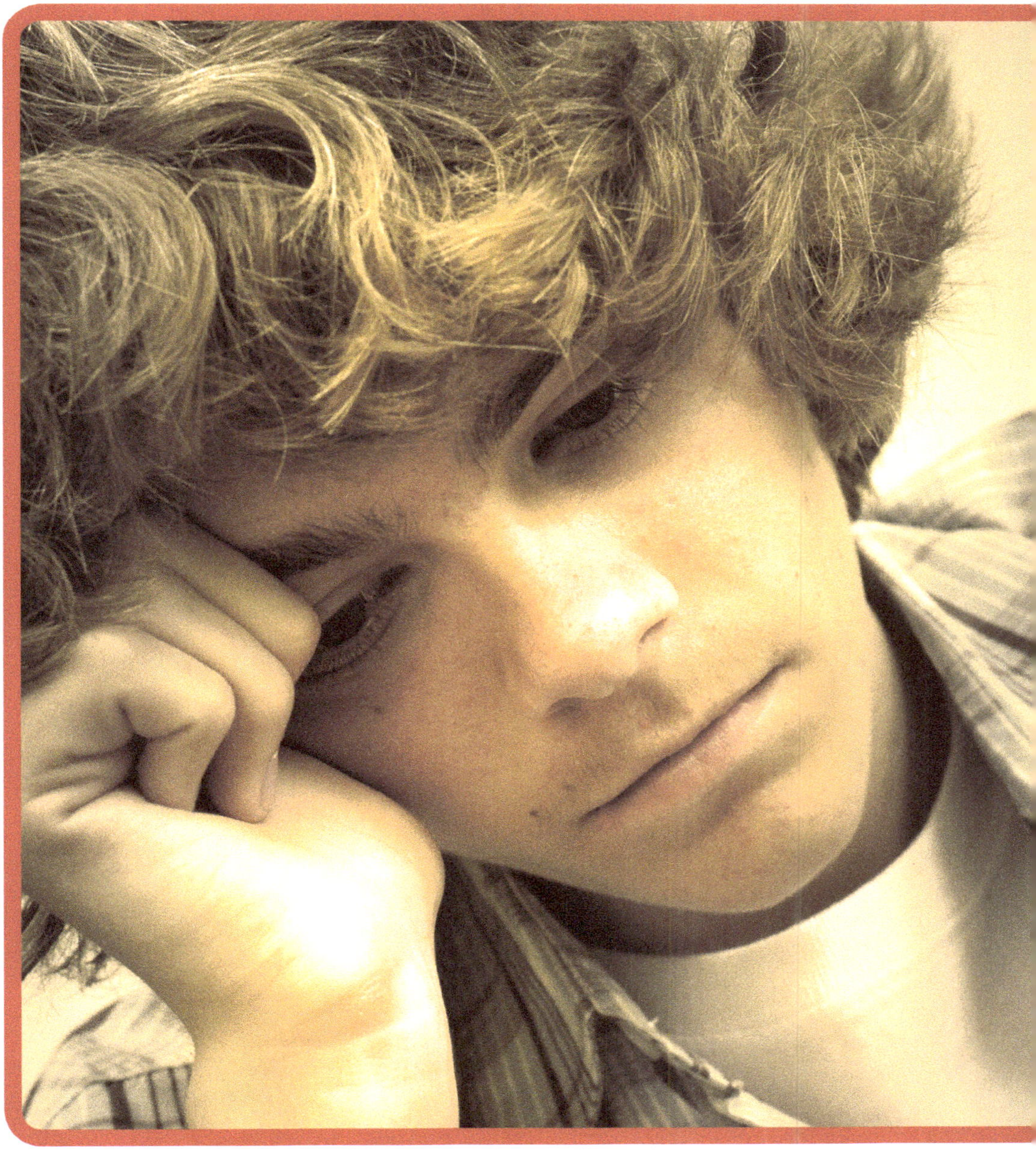

An unhappy teen appears lost in thought. Inhalant use may cause sadness or loss of interest in friends and school. Habitual inhalant use may result in behavioral issues or depression.

nasal passages and may develop infections in the throat and ear. Habitual inhalant users often have low energy, experience sleep problems, and lose weight. They may appear anxious, excitable, or irritable, even when they have not used an inhalant recently.

Specific inhalants are linked to particular damages to the body. Dry-cleaning fluids and solvents containing toluene may cause liver and kidney damage. Trichloroethylene, found in degreasers and spot removers, can lead to cirrhosis of the liver and damage to hearing and vision. Methylene chloride, which is

THE HAZARDS OF CANNED AIR

People use products sold as "canned air" to remove dust from computers and other electronic equipment. Some people also abuse these products, using them as inhalants. Although these products sound safe, they contain dangerous chemicals rather than air.

Some canned air products, particularly those containing difluoroethane, are flammable. People abusing these products, as well as those using them as intended, have been burned when the chemicals caught fire. The chemicals in canned air cool quickly when released from the can. Abusers may suffer frostbite when the frigid gas from canned air comes into contact with skin and other parts of the body. Prolonged exposure to canned air may lead to serious frostbite, resulting in damage to nerves, muscles, and other tissues. Inhaling canned air can also cause suffocation because the fumes keep oxygen from entering the lungs. Researchers believe that habitual use of canned air as an inhalant can damage nerves in the nervous system.

found in varnish and paint thinners, affects the heart and heartbeat. Repeated use of some inhalants, particularly spray paint, may cause permanent lung damage.

Benzene, which is found in gasoline, may injure red blood cells, which may interfere with the supply of oxygen to body cells. Benzene may also weaken the body's immune system by damaging bone marrow, which produces white blood cells. Having fewer white blood cells makes a person more susceptible to colds and other infections and diseases. The use of hexane, an ingredient in glue and gasoline, causes damage to the peripheral nervous system. The nerves carrying messages to and from the spinal cord stop working properly.

Propane and butane—a gas found in lighter fluid and such aerosols as spray paint and hair spray—are highly flammable. If they catch fire during use, serious burns or other injuries may occur. Repeated use of nitrous oxide may lead to spasms in arms and legs and a loss of sensation in various body parts.

Long-term use of nitrites can lead to persistent high blood pressure and heart disease. Research on animals has shown possible links between nitrite use and an increased risk of cancer and an increased risk of damage to the user's immune system. Older teens and adults who use nitrites usually inhale them to enhance their sexual experiences. Research has shown a link between the abuse of nitrites and unsafe sex. Abusers of nitrites sometimes fail to use safe-sex methods when high on nitrites. Unsafe sex can lead to pregnancy or the spread of HIV/AIDS, hepatitis, and other infectious diseases.

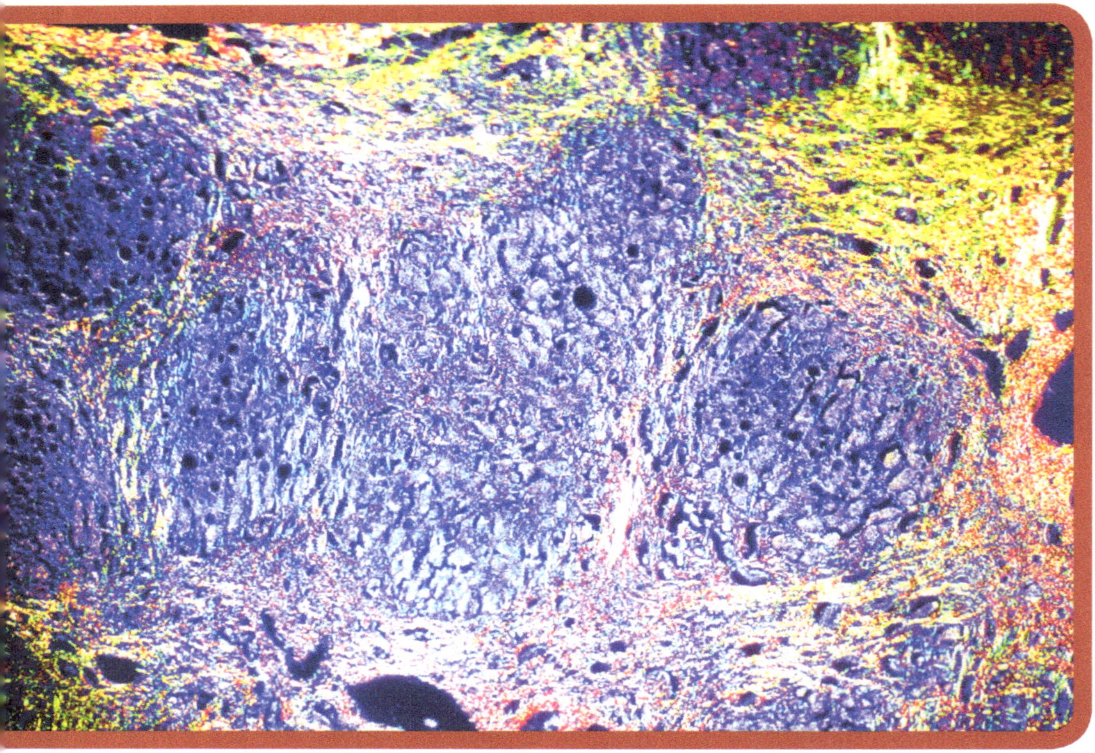

The yellow and red areas in this image are scar tissue in a liver damaged by cirrhosis. Long-term use of spot removers or degreasers as an inhalant can result in cirrhosis of the liver.

Using inhalants during pregnancy can harm a developing fetus. The chemicals in inhalants can reduce birth weight, cause skeletal and nervous system abnormalities, and impair a child's development. Research has shown that the children of mothers who abuse solvents, especially those containing toluene, have symptoms similar to children suffering from fetal alcohol syndrome.

Death and Injuries

Inhalant use can kill. The most common cause of death from using inhalants is known as sudden sniffing death syndrome. When a person inhales the highly concentrated chemicals in most solvents and aerosols, the chemicals make the heart beat rapidly and irregularly. The stress to the heart sometimes causes the heart to suddenly stop beating. Cardiac arrest, or heart failure, can result within minutes after using an inhalant, even if the person is healthy. Some young people have died from sudden sniffing death syndrome the very first time they experimented with an inhalant.

Sniffing inhalants from a plastic or paper bag can cause death by suffocation. The bag prevents oxygen from reaching the lungs. A person may also suffocate when the fumes from an inhalant fill the lungs, preventing them from absorbing oxygen. Inhalant users sometimes vomit after sniffing or huffing. Some have died from choking on their own vomit.

Some users have suffered serious or fatal injuries while intoxicated on inhalants. The impairment of brain functioning during an inhalant high often leads users to make poor decisions. They may crash a car or bike while impaired. They may do reckless things, such as jumping off a building or starting a fire. Some inhalant users become aggressive while buzzed and may start fights with other people. Inhalant users also may not notice that they are in a dangerous situation, such as wandering into traffic on a busy street or having trouble staying afloat in a pool.

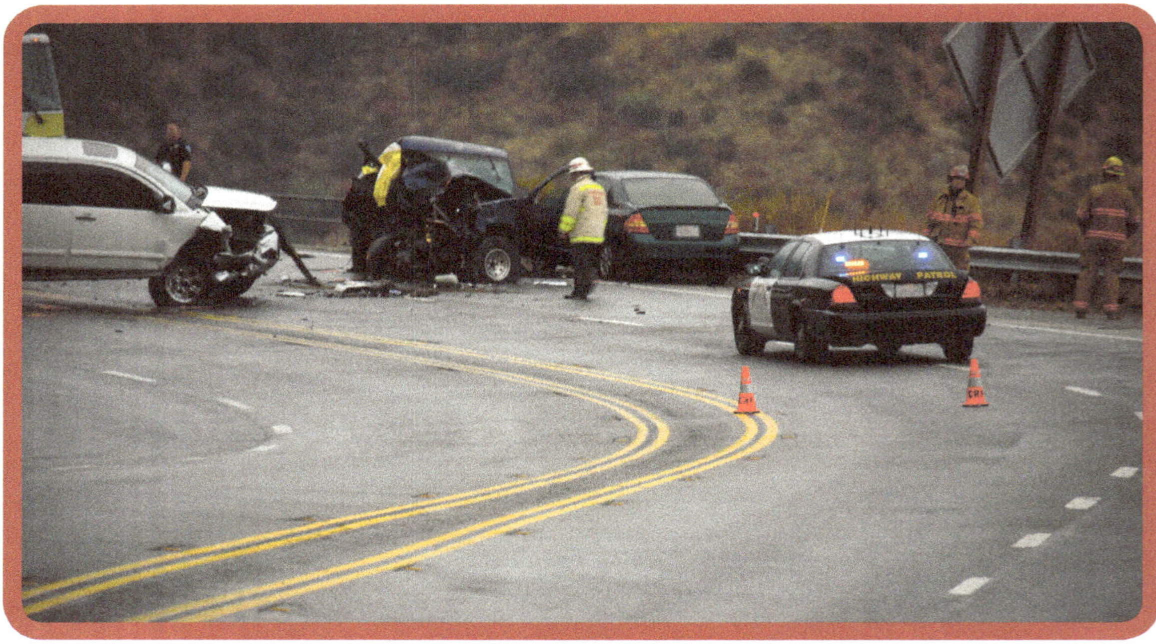

Emergency responders work at the scene of a fatal car accident. An inhalant user's judgment and coordination may be impaired, making it dangerous for that person to drive or perform other activities.

Some long-term inhalant users become depressed. They become apathetic, meaning that they do not want to do anything and care about nothing. They start skipping classes, getting failing grades, and experiencing other problems at school. They may get into arguments with family and friends. They may lose friends and start hanging around only with other inhalant users. Depression may also lead a habitual inhalant user to commit suicide.

CHAPTER 4

ADDICTED TO HUFFING

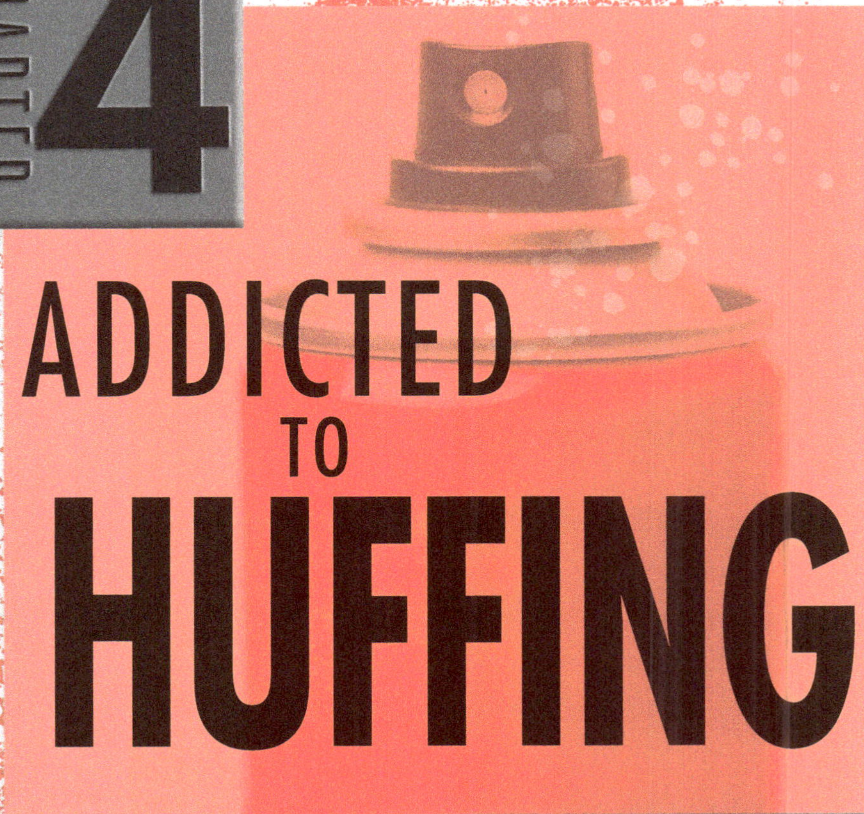

Because inhalants are widely available, they are a common choice for first-time or younger drug users seeking a quick, cheap high. Inhalants are simpler to obtain, and inhalant use is often easier to conceal from parents, friends, and other people than the use of most other drugs. So users may be able to continue huffing for long periods of time before their use of inhalants is noticed.

The damage caused by the long-term use of inhalants may appear gradually. The toxic chemicals slowly accumulate in the brain and body, and users often do not realize that they are physically harming themselves. Because inhalants affect brain functioning, users may also not have the mental ability to recognize the obvious signs of drug addiction.

The Basics of Addiction

Addiction occurs when a person has a strong need for something. A person can become addicted to many drugs, including alcohol, the nicotine in cigarettes, and both illegal and prescription drugs. People also become addicted to activities, such as gambling, shopping, or surfing the Internet. These substances and behaviors provide the user pleasure or a temporary escape from the stresses and problems of life. Sometimes the need for the drug or activity becomes overwhelming and eventually disrupts the user's life.

A person has an addiction when he or she becomes dependent on a drug. An addict cannot function normally without using an abused drug. Most drug users who develop a dependency show several signs. They start to feel a compulsion, or irresistible craving, to use the drug. Obtaining and using a drug becomes the primary focus of an addict's life. They also begin suffering from withdrawal symptoms when they stop using the drug, either by choice or because they do not have a supply of the drug. An addict will start using the drug to avoid the withdrawal symptoms, rather than experience the high or escape that the drug provides.

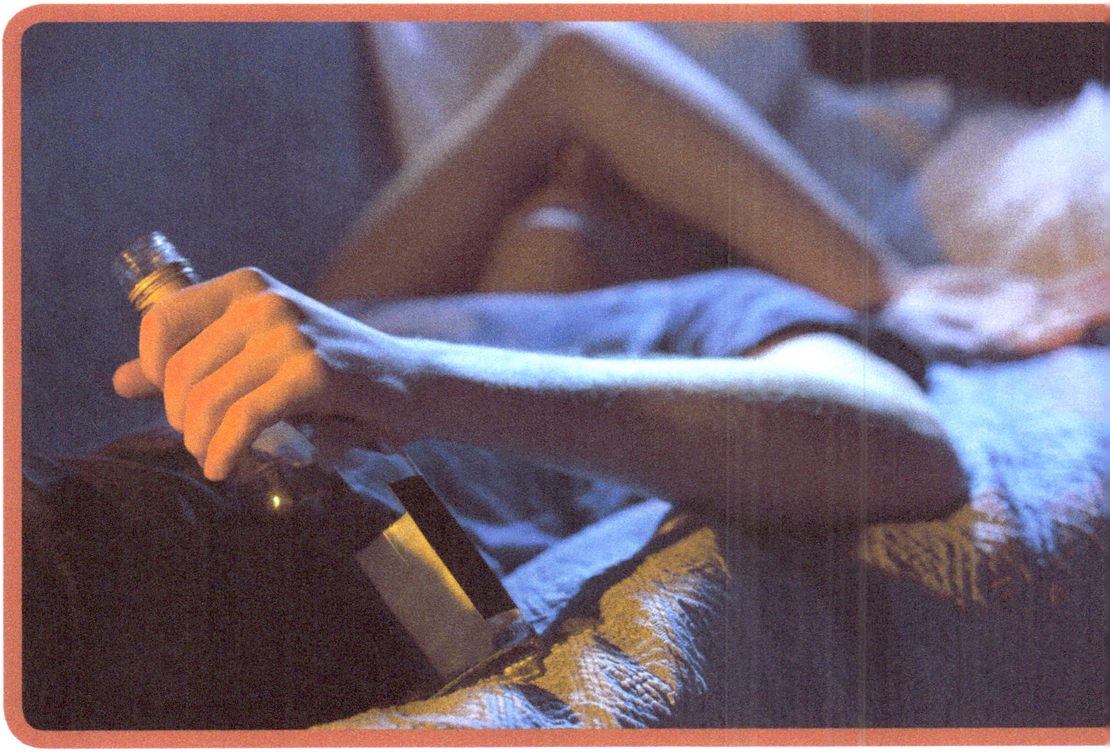

A teen suffering from an addiction to alcohol clutches an empty liquor bottle. An addiction to inhalants, like an alcohol addiction, produces an overwhelming desire to use the drug.

Drug tolerance is an important factor in drug dependence. When a person first takes a drug, the substance changes the way the body keeps its systems in balance. Over time, the body adapts to the regular use of a drug. The person develops what is known as a tolerance to a drug. To experience the same high to which he or she is accustomed, a drug user must use increasingly larger, more frequent, or more powerful doses of the drug.

Drug addiction has two distinct elements. Physical addiction is a biological condition in which the addict's body develops a physical dependence on a drug. When the person stops using the drug, he or she suffers a physical reaction known as withdrawal. For some drugs, withdrawal symptoms are mild or unnoticeable. The withdrawal symptoms of other drugs, such as heroin and alcohol, can be severe or even fatal. Psychological addiction is an emotional or mental urge to keep using a drug. A drug user feels that the drug is necessary to maintain a normal life. For instance, a person with a psychological addiction will instinctively use a drug when distressed or in a particular setting, even when he or she does not experience withdrawal

INHALANT WITHDRAWAL SYMPTOMS

When a habitual user stops using an inhalant, he or she may suffer a variety of withdrawal symptoms. Physical symptoms include excessive sweating, fast heartbeat, nausea, muscle aches, hand tremors, and severe headache. The person may also feel weak or tired, sleep excessively, and experience vivid dreams or hallucinations. Emotional symptoms linked to withdrawal include depression, anxiety, restlessness, and aggressiveness. In severe cases, withdrawal from inhalant use can cause convulsions.

symptoms due to a physical addiction. The stress or setting triggers the person's drug use. Most drug addictions involve both physical and psychological elements.

Addiction to Inhalants

All inhalants are psychologically addictive. The intoxicating effect of most inhalants occurs because they slow down the brain and nervous system. In research studies, inhalant users have reported that they experienced a strong urge to keep using inhalants because they felt they needed them to function normally. This urge appears to occur most often when a person has been using inhalants regularly over many consecutive days. A compulsive craving to use inhalants indicates that a psychological dependency has developed.

Some inhalants appear to cause a physical dependency. Research has shown that some inhalants, particularly those containing toluene, trigger an increase in the activity of dopamine. Dopamine is a natural chemical that plays a key role in the brain's reward system. Studies have revealed that dopamine makes it possible for the brain to recognize potential pleasure, joy, or satisfaction experiences and to take action to obtain these rewards. When dopamine activity in the brain rises, a person feels a greater sense of well-being. Long-term disruption of the dopamine system is often a factor in drug addiction. An addict becomes dependent on the sense of well-being produced when a drug, including an inhalant, is used.

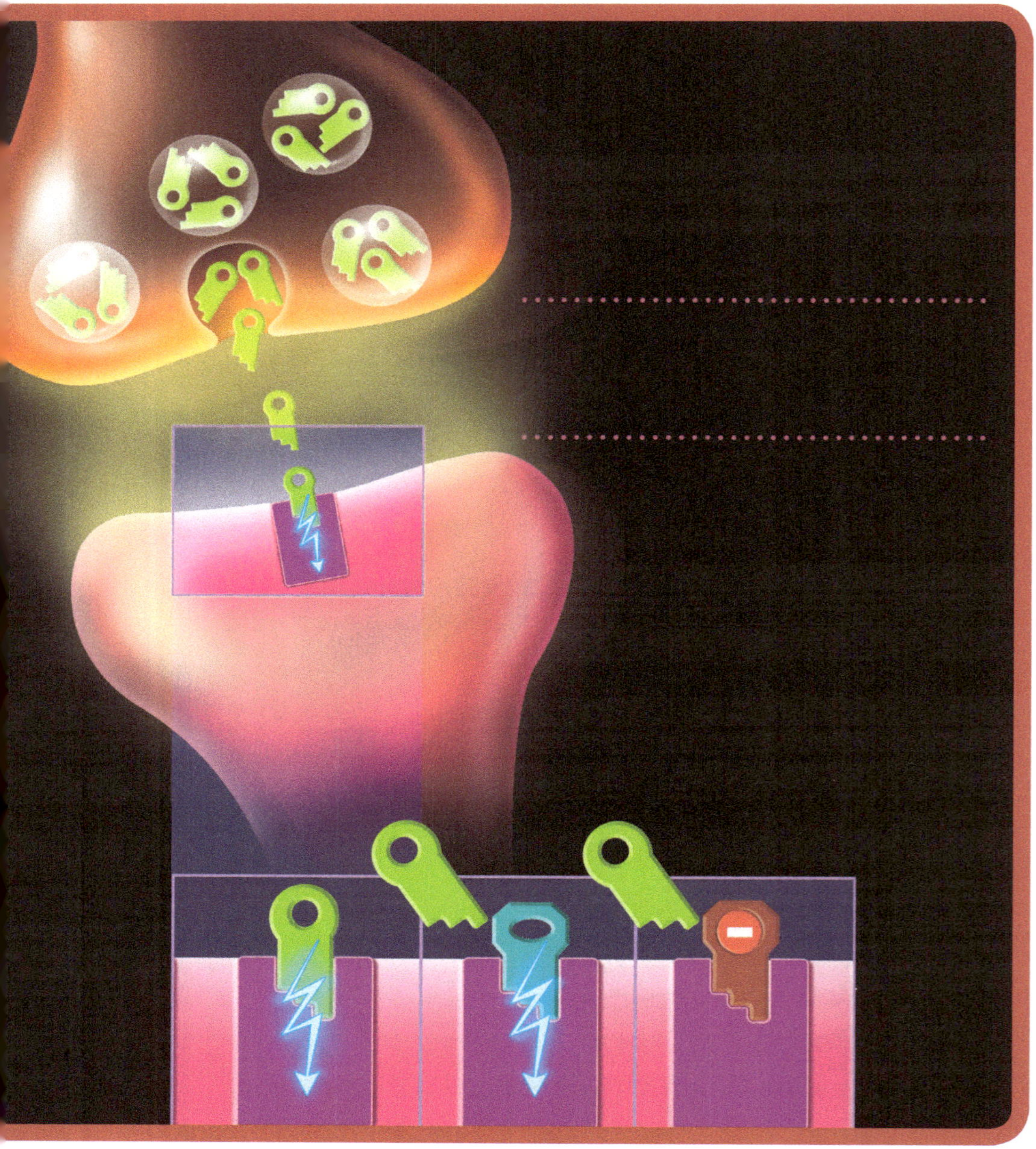

This illustration shows how dopamine transmission works. When the brain releases dopamine *(green key)*, it can link only with a receptor neuron *(bottom left)* associated with pleasure. Multiple linkages allow the nerve impulse to travel along neural networks and result in pleasurable feelings. Long-term inhalant use can impair dopamine transmission.

The pathway to an inhalant addiction is the same for most users. Inhalants have only a temporary effect, which leads to repeated use over a short period of time to prolong the high. Eventually, a user cannot stop thinking about inhaling and cannot live without the high for long periods. If a habitual user tries to stop inhaling, he or she experiences withdrawal symptoms. Withdrawal symptoms sometimes occur as soon as twenty-four hours after the last inhalant use. One study showed that about half of the subjects who were dependent on inhalants reported significant withdrawal symptoms.

Signs of Inhalant Abuse and Addiction

Most inhalants produce only short-term intoxicating effects, so infrequent users may be able to conceal their use because they appear normal soon after using an inhalant. Habitual users, however, begin to display certain physical signs and behaviors that indicate they are abusing inhalants. The physical signs of frequent inhalant abuse include slurred or confused speech and a lack of physical coordination. Habitual users may also have rashes or blisters on their faces, frequently have a runny nose and cough, and their eyes may be watery or their pupils may be dilated. They may vomit frequently or have extremely bad breath that smells like chemicals.

Habitual inhalant users may appear drunk, dazed, or dizzy much of the time. They may complain about being tired and may have no appetite. Excessive weight loss is a frequent

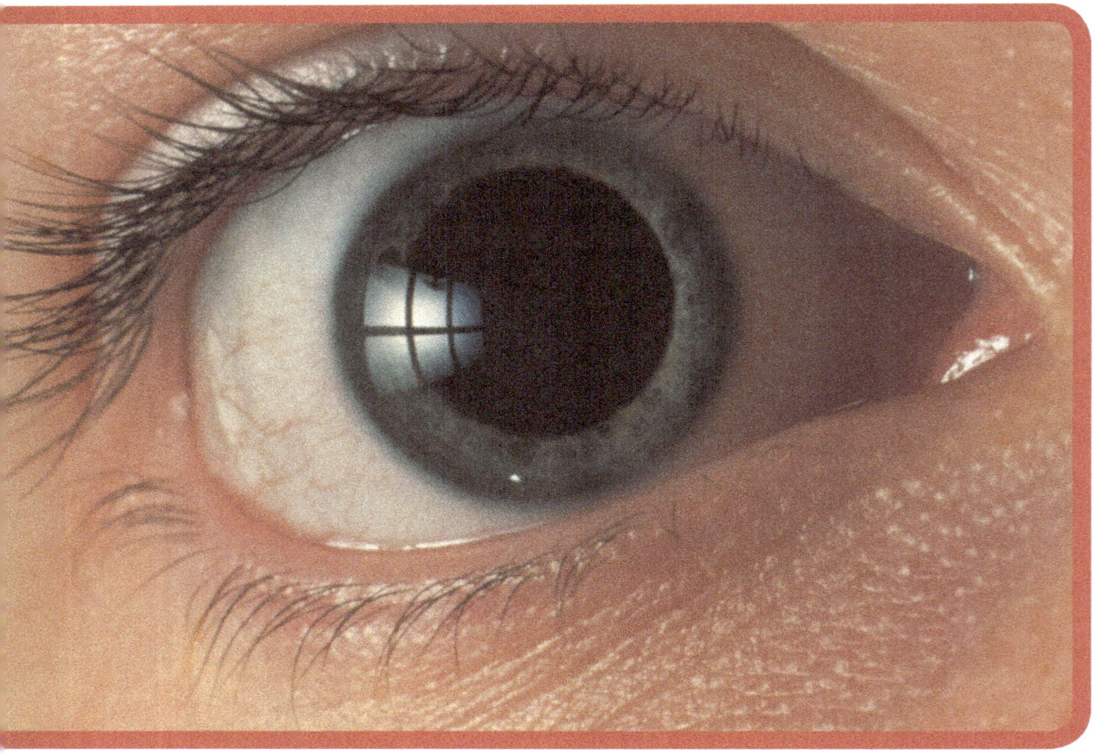

This close-up photo shows a dilated pupil in the center of an eye. Perceiving that a person is abusing inhalants is difficult, but long-term abusers sometimes have dilated pupils even in bright light.

consequence of habitual inhalant abuse. Inhalant abusers may also display abrupt mood changes, swinging from happy to sad or intense to disinterested. They may seem anxious, excitable, restless, irritable, or angry.

Inhalant abusers may have paint or other substances on their face, lips, nose, or other body parts. They may paint their fingernails with certain inhalants, such as marker pens or correction fluid, so that they can sniff the substances whenever they want. Inhalant abusers may constantly smell their clothes—particularly collars, sleeves, or hair scrunchies—where they have applied substances to be inhaled. They may have an unusual amount of markers, lighters, correction fluid, or other often abused products in their room, backpack, or locker.

Parents may notice that household products are missing. They may find rags, cloths, or other items used in the inhaling process hidden around the house. Family members may notice that an abuser is neglecting his or her appearance or aggressively tries to prevent family members from entering his or her room, where inhalants may be stashed. An abuser may suddenly start having problems at school.

TEN GREAT QUESTIONS TO ASK A DRUG COUNSELOR

1. If I use inhalants only once in a while, can I become addicted?
2. What are the potential damages caused by the inhalant(s) I have used?
3. Are any of these damages permanent?
4. What are the signs of inhalant addiction?
5. What do I need to do to stop using inhalants?
6. If I stop using inhalants, what withdrawal symptoms will I experience?
7. Should I tell my parents about my problem with inhalants?
8. Is there a nearby treatment program or facility that can help me stop using inhalants?
9. Can you recommend a therapist who can help me with my recovery?
10. How can I help my friends who continue to huff?

CHAPTER 5

FINDING HELP

When you're addicted to an inhalant, you cannot control your drug use. You continue using the inhalant despite the harm it causes. You may want to quit, but habitual users of inhalants find they cannot do it on their own. You will need help from your doctor, family, or an organized treatment program to overcome your addiction to inhalants and stay off them for good.

Behavioral Treatment

A variety of treatments help people overcome their drug addiction. The two main methods are treating a person with medications and using behavioral treatments. Almost all treatment programs for inhalant addiction are the behavioral type. Medications are generally prescribed only to help an addict who has stopped using inhalants handle the withdrawal symptoms that he or she is experiencing.

People who use inhalants have different characteristics from those who abuse most other drugs. Inhalant abusers sometimes have low self-esteem or are involved in difficult family situations. As a result of inhalant use, they may be disinterested in most things, so it may be difficult to motivate them to participate in a drug treatment program. The chemicals in inhalants may have impaired their brains, making it difficult for them to make sound treatment decisions and stick with a treatment plan. Inhalant abusers and addicts commonly use more than one drug. Because of these various factors, treatment for inhalant abusers is often more complex.

To overcome an addiction to inhalants, a person must stay away from them. For most abusers, this means getting around-the-clock treatment in a drug treatment facility. Because inhalant abuse creates a psychological dependence—and in some cases, a physical dependence—counselors at a treatment facility teach addicts how to control their cravings for inhalants. They also help addicts get through the withdrawal stage.

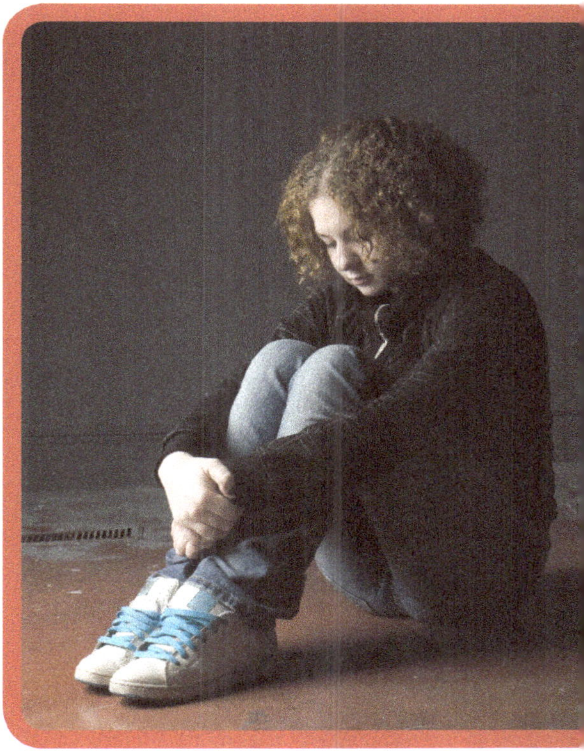

A long-term inhalant abuser is often apathetic and passive, which makes it difficult to convince him or her to enter into an addiction treatment program.

The primary method of treating an inhalant addiction is to convince an addict that his or her life is better when not using inhalants. This method is known as behavioral treatment, or behavioral-change intervention. The goal of behavioral treatment is to provide inhalant abusers with the ability to change the behavioral patterns related to their drug abuse and stick to their new behavioral patterns in the future.

Detoxification

For an inhalant abuser seeking help, the first step in the recovery process is detoxification. The toxic chemicals in inhalants build up in the body of a habitual user. Detoxification is the process of cleaning these chemicals out of the body. Detoxification works only if the person stops using inhalants completely. Users often abuse more than one inhalant, so the staff members at a treatment facility will identify the specific substances used by taking a detailed history of the abuser's inhalant use. They also conduct a thorough physical examination to determine the presence of any physical effects from inhalant use. If the abuser has any medical problems, the facility will provide medical care.

Rehabilitation

Once an addict gets through the detoxification stage, he or she enters a longer-term drug behavioral rehabilitation program.

WHEN SOMEONE YOU KNOW IS USING INHALANTS

If you have a family member or friend who is using inhalants, it will not be easy for the person to stop using them. You may be able to help the person by talking to and offering to assist him or her. The first step is to tell the user you care about him or her and ask why he or she is using inhalants. Listen to the user and encourage him or her to try to stop using inhalants. Avoid criticizing the person's behavior and choices because drug users often become defensive when they are attacked over their drug use. Ask the user how you can help and urge him or her to participate in common activities with family and friends. Try to convince the user to stop hanging around with people you suspect are using inhalants with him or her. If the person starts using inhalants again after ceasing for a while, do not show frustration or anger. Tell the individual that you know giving it up is not easy and encourage him or her to try to stop again. Remember that when someone is addicted to a drug, the only person who can decide to stop using is the addict.

Some rehab facilities provide residential programs, meaning that the person lives at the rehab facility for a certain period of time, often a month or two, usually without ever leaving the facility. In this safe setting, the user can focus all of his or her attention and efforts on recovering from the addiction to inhalants. Most important, the addict is completely cut off from access to inhalants while at the facility or kept away from them when outside the facility.

A rehab facility provides individual and family counseling, as well as education on inhalants and other drugs. Its staff also provides group counseling, although inhalant users are often slowly and carefully introduced into some group counseling settings. People addicted to other types of drugs are usually older than typical inhalant users and tend to look down on them or tease them. They frequently view inhalant abusers as uncool, foolish, immature, or unsophisticated. Rehab programs also teach recovering addicts how to develop positive habits, such as eating healthy foods and exercising regularly.

Once an inhalant abuser has demonstrated that he or she is in control of the addiction, counselors at a rehab facility will help that individual develop a long-term recovery plan. They will also help a recovering addict prepare to return to his or her life before the inhalant addiction took over. Counselors will refer a recovering addict to self-help groups in the community and introduce him or her to school or work programs and other resources that can help the person successfully adjust to his or her new life. Aftercare groups help provide ongoing recovery support once a recovering addict leaves a rehab facility. Meeting with other people recovering from an inhalant addiction, as well as people recovering from other drug addictions, helps a recovering addict avoid returning to drug use.

Outpatient drug rehabilitation programs offer more flexibility than residential treatment programs. Outpatient programs meet several times a week, usually at night. Participation in an outpatient program allows inhalant abusers to continue living at home while overcoming their addiction. Outpatient treatment programs can be ineffective for many inhalant abusers, mainly because an outpatient program, unlike a residential program, does not wall off an abuser from easy access to inhalants. Because of the widespread availability of inhalants, an abuser is likely to come into contact again with inhalants during daily life at home, work, or school. The temptation to start using an inhalant may be too great to resist for an abuser in an outpatient program.

Another factor that helps inhalant addicts recover is improving the bond between them and their parents. In some cases, parents of inhalant addicts may need guidance to improve their parenting skills. Aftercare counselors and parents should encourage and help a recovering inhalant abuser find new friends who do not abuse inhalants or other drugs. Introducing recovering inhalant abusers to safe and healthy types of recreation and other activities has proved to be an effective method to help an inhalant abuser devote his energies to behaviors other than drug use.

Preventing Relapse

The most important aspect of behavioral treatment for inhalant addiction is to prevent relapses. A relapse is a return to a regular pattern of drug use. A single drug-use event is often called a "lapse." The difference between a relapse and a lapse can be important. A lapse may only require counseling to get a recovering addict back on track. A relapse may be more complicated, especially if it rekindles a physical dependence on inhalants.

Relapse is a common problem for inhalant addicts because the psychological need that they feel for inhalants remains very

FINDING A TREATMENT CENTER

It may be challenging to find a treatment center near you that provides help for inhalant abusers. Many drug treatment facilities do not accept inhalant addicts because they do not admit teenagers to their programs or because they lack expertise in dealing with inhalant addiction. If you or a friend needs help for inhalant abuse, contact the National Inhalant Prevention Coalition at (800) 269-4237. The organization can provide general information on inhalants and addiction treatments and help you find a treatment center in your area that admits inhalant abusers. The Substance Abuse and Mental Health Services Administration's treatment referral helpline at (800) 662-HELP also offers assistance to those seeking a treatment center for inhalant abuse.

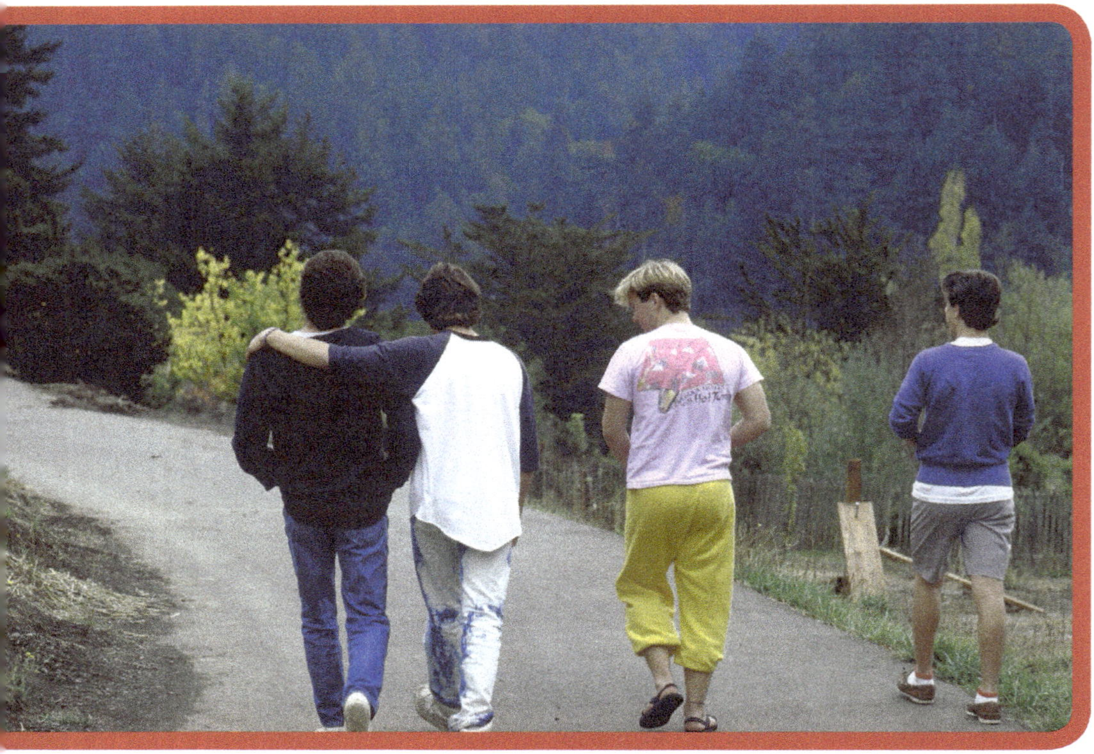

Four teens in a drug treatment program take a stroll at a rural treatment facility. Support from other drug abusers can help inhalant addicts overcome their addiction and avoid relapse.

strong. Another factor that contributes to a high rate of relapse among inhalant abusers is that completing a treatment program, they will often come into contact with products that can be abused as an inhalant. Aftercare programs are a crucial part of preventing relapse in an inhalant abuser. An inhalant abuser may need counseling and the support supplied by group meetings for as many as two years before fully recovering.

Admitting That You Have a Problem

The first step to getting help for inhalant abuse is admitting that you have a problem. You have a problem with inhalants if you feel that you must use inhalants regularly or need the drug to deal with life. You have a problem if you are spending increasing amounts of your time and efforts obtaining inhalants or if you are stealing inhalants or spending lots of money to buy them. You have a problem if you engage in dangerous activities when you are high on inhalants. You have a problem if you tried to stop using inhalants, but your cravings are too strong and you go back to using them again.

If you think you or a friend may be addicted to inhalants, seek help. It is extremely challenging to overcome an inhalant addiction by yourself. If you are reluctant to approach a parent, talk to your doctor, a counselor or nurse at your school, or another trusted adult. One of them can help you find the medical care, counseling, education, and long-term support that you need to treat your addiction.

GLOSSARY

acute Having a severe and sudden onset of a condition, in which symptoms appear and change or worsen rapidly.

addiction A physical or psychological need to use a drug, resulting in withdrawal symptoms if the drug is not taken.

chronic Having a long-developing condition, in which the condition progresses and worsens over an extended period of time.

depression A deep feeling of sadness, particularly one that persists.

detoxification A process in which the body rids itself of a drug.

huffing The act of inhaling a substance for the purpose of getting high.

neuron A special type of nerve cell in the brain and body that processes and transmits information.

rehabilitation A program of medical care, psychological treatment, and education that helps an addict overcome dependency on a drug.

tolerance A condition in which a drug user needs a higher dose of a drug to produce the same effect experienced during early uses of the drug.

withdrawal Symptoms that occur when someone with a drug addiction abruptly stops or reduces drug use.

FOR MORE INFORMATION

American Association of Poison Control Centers (AAPCC)
515 King Street, Suite 510
Alexandria, VA 22314
(703) 894-1858; Help Line (800) 222-1222
Web site: http://www.aapcc.org
The AAPCC's poison centers offer free and private medical advice twenty-four hours a day, every day.

Canadian Centre on Substance Abuse
75 Albert Street, Suite 500
Ottawa, ON K1P 5E7
Canada
(613) 235-4048
Web site: http://www.ccsa.ca
This Canadian governmental agency provides information on inhalants and other drug abuse issues.

National Institute on Drug Abuse (NIDA)
6001 Executive Boulevard, Room 5213
Bethesda, MD 20892-9561
(301) 443-1124
Web site: http://www.drugabuse.gov
This U.S. government research institute provides comprehensive information on drugs, including how they affect the brain and the body.

National Inhalant Prevention Coalition (NIPC)
318 Lindsay Street
Chattanooga, TN 37403
(800) 269-4237
Web site: http://www.inhalants.org
The NIPC provides a wide range of information on inhalants, inhalant abuse, and prevention programs.

Substance Abuse and Mental Health Services Administration (SAMHSA)
P.O. Box 2345
Rockville, MD 20847-2345
(877) 726-4727
Web site: http://www.samhsa.gov
This agency provides information on drug abuse, including a database on treatment facilities.

Web Sites

Due to the changing nature of Internet links, Rosen Publishing has developed an online list of Web sites related to the subject of this book. This site is updated regularly. Please use this link to access the list:

http://www.rosenlinks.com/DAC/Inhal

FOR FURTHER READING

D'Souza, Barnabe. *From Ecstasy to Agony and Back: Journeying with Adolescents on the Street.* Thousand Oaks, CA: Sage, 2012.

Fisher, Gary L., and Nancy A. Roget, eds. *Encyclopedia of Substance Abuse Prevention, Treatment, and Recovery.* Thousand Oaks, CA: Sage, 2008.

Fletcher, Anne M. *Inside Rehab: The Surprising Truth About Addiction Treatment—and How to Get Help That Works.* New York, NY: Viking, 2013.

Flynn, Noa. *Inhalants and Solvents: Sniffing Disaster.* Greensboro, NC: Mason Crest, 2012.

Hollen, Kathryn H. *Encyclopedia of Addictions.* Santa Barbara, CA: Greenwood, 2008.

National Institute on Drug Abuse. *Drugs, Brains, and Behavior: The Science of Addiction.* Bethesda, MD: NIDA, 2010.

National Institute on Drug Abuse. *Seeking Drug Abuse Treatment: Know What to Ask.* Bethesda, MD: NIDA, 2011.

Sheff, Nic. *We All Fall Down: Living with Addiction.* New York, NY: Little, Brown, 2011.

Sweeney, Michael S. *Brain: The Complete Mind: How It Develops, How It Works, and How to Keep It Sharp.* Washington, DC: National Geographic, 2009.

U.S. Drug Enforcement Agency. *Drugs of Abuse.* Washington, DC: 2011.

BIBLIOGRAPHY

Canadian Centre on Substance Abuse. "Designing a Tool to Measure the Impact of Client Length of Stay on Treatment Outcome." Retrieved April 11, 2013 (http://www.ccsa.ca/2005%20CCSA%20Documents/ccsa-011138-2005.pdf).

Foundation for a Drug Free World. "The Truth About Inhalants." Retrieved on April 8, 2013 (http://www.drugfreeworld.org/drugfacts/inhalants.html).

Genesis House. "Inhalant Addiction." Retrieved April 9, 2013 (http://www.genesishouse.net/article-Inhalant-Addiction.html).

Johnston, L. D., P. M. O'Malley, J. G. Bachman, and J. E. Schulenberg. *Monitoring the Future National Results on Drug Use: 2012 Overview, Key Findings on Adolescent Drug Use*. Ann Arbor, MI: Institute for Social Research, The University of Michigan, 2013. Retrieved April 9, 2013 (http://www.monitoringthefuture.org/pubs/monographs/mtf-overview2012.pdf).

Mayo Clinic. "Drug Addiction." Retrieved April 9, 2013 (http://www.mayoclinic.com/health/drug-addiction/DS00183).

National Highway Traffic Safety Administration. "Drugs and Human Performance Fact Sheets: Toluene." Retrieved April 10, 2013 (http://www.nhtsa.gov/people/injury/research/job185drugs/toluene.htm).

National Institute of Mental Health. "Brain Basics." Retrieved April 8, 2013 (http://www.nimh.nih.gov/health/educational-resources/brain-basics/brain-basics.shtml).

National Institute on Drug Abuse. "Inhalant Abuse: A Volatile Research Agenda." Retrieved April 9, 2013 (http://archives.drugabuse.gov/pdf/monographs/129.pdf).

State of Colorado. "Colorado Revised Statue 18-18-412 (2)." Retrieved April 11, 2013 (http://www.colorado.gov/cs/Satellite?blobcol=urldata&blobheader=application%2Fpdf&blobkey=id&blobtable=MungoBlobs&blobwhere=1251704777335&ssbinary=true).

Substance Abuse and Mental Health Services Administration. "Substance Abuse Treatment Advisory: Inhalants." Retrieved April 11, 1013 (http://kap.samhsa.gov/products/manuals/advisory/pdfs/Inhalants-Advisory.pdf).

Substance Abuse and Mental Health Services Administration. "Results from the 2011 National Survey on Drug Use and Health: Illicit Drug Use Tables 1.1 to 1.92." Retrieved April 9, 2013 (http://www.samhsa.gov/data/NSDUH/2011SummNatFindDetTables/NSDUH-DetTabsPDFWHTML2011/2k11DetailedTabs/Web/HTML/NSDUH-DetTabsSect1peTabs1to46-2011.htm)

Washington State Department of Labor and Industries. "Improper Use of Canned-Air Products Can Cause Flash Fires and Injury." Retrieved April 10, 2013 (http://www.lni.wa.gov/Safety/Basics/HazAlerts/CannedAir0608.asp).

INDEX

About the Author

G. S. Prentzas is an author and editor who has written more than thirty books for young readers, including *The World Health Organization*, and edited medical textbooks. He graduated from the University of North Carolina with an A.B.; with honors in English and a J.D. with honors.

Photo Credits

Cover, p. 1 Swettlana Gordacheva/Shutterstock.com; pp. 4–5 Sinisa Botas/Shutterstock.com; pp. 8, 19, 28, 37, 47, 56, 57, 59, 60, 62 Elena Agibalova/Shutterstock.com; p. 9 Nata-Lia/ Shutterstock.com; p. 11 Charles D Winters/Photo Researchers/ Getty Images; p. 14 SPL/Science Source; p. 15 Brand X Pictures/Thinkstock; pp. 21, 25 National Institute on Drug Abuse (NIDA)/NIH; pp. 23, 36 iStockphoto/Thinkstock; p. 31 Junial Enterprises/Shutterstock.com; p. 34 Cultura Science/ Michael J. Klein, M.D./Oxford Scientific/Getty Images; p. 39 Stokkete/Shutterstock.com; p. 42 BSIP/Universal Images Group/ Getty Images; p. 44 Adam Hart-Davis/Science Source; p. 49 @ erics/Shutterstock.com; p. 54 Matthew Naythons/Time & Life Pictures/Getty Images.

Designer: Sam Zavieh; Editor: Kathy Kuhtz Campbell;
Photo Researcher: Marty Levick